Acid Reflux Cookbook

Overcome GERD and LPR with Flavorful, Gluten-Free Recipes and a Comprehensive 30-Day Plan for Lasting Relief and Vibrant Health

Peter S. Benson

Copyright © 2024 by Peter S. Benson

All rights reserved
No part of this publication may be reproduced, stored in a retrieval system. or transmitted. in and form or by any means, electronic, mechanical, photocopying, recording, or otherwise, without the prior written permission of the author.
The information in this ebook is true and complete to the best of our knowledge. All recommendations are made without guarantee on the part of the author or publisher. The author and publisher disclaim any liability in connection with the use of this information.

Table of Contents

Acid Reflux Cookbook 1

Introduction 6

Chapter 1: Understanding Acid Reflux 8

    What is Acid Reflux? 8

    Causes and Triggers of Acid Reflux 10

    Symptoms of Acid Reflux 12

    Complications of Untreated Acid Reflux 14

Chapter 2: Managing Acid Reflux Through Diet 17

    The Role of Diet in Acid Reflux Management 17

    Foods to Avoid for Acid Reflux 20

    Foods that May Help Alleviate Acid Reflux Symptoms 22

    Tips for Eating and Drinking to Prevent Acid Reflux 24

Chapter 3: Meal Planning for Acid Reflux 27

    Principles of Acid Reflux-Friendly Meal Planning 27

    Sample Meal Plans for Breakfast, Lunch, and Dinner 30

    Snack Ideas for Acid Reflux Relief 32

Chapter 4: Acid Reflux Friendly Recipes 34

    Breakfast Recipes 34

    Oatmeal with Bananas and Almonds 34

    Greek Yogurt Parfait with Berries 36

    Egg White Veggie Omelet 38

    Lunch Recipes 41

    Quinoa Salad with Grilled Chicken 41

Turkey and Avocado Wrap 44

Salmon and Vegetable Stir-Fry 46

Dinner Recipes 49

Baked Chicken Breast with Roasted Vegetables 49

Shrimp and Vegetable Skewers 52

Vegetable and Lentil Soup 54

Snack Recipes 57

Almond Butter and Banana Rice Cakes 57

Greek Yogurt with Honey and Almonds 59

Cucumber and Hummus Snack Platter 61

Chapter 5: Beverages for Acid Reflux Relief 63

Herbal Teas for Soothing Acid Reflux 63

Non-Acidic Fruit and Vegetable Juices 66

Infused Water Recipes for Hydration 68

Chapter 6: Desserts and Treats for Acid Reflux 71

Banana Ice Cream 71

Baked Apples with Cinnamon 73

Mango Coconut Chia Pudding 75

Chapter 7: Tips for Dining Out with Acid Reflux 77

Choosing Acid Reflux-Friendly Restaurants 77

Strategies for Ordering Acid Reflux-Friendly Meals 80

Handling Social Situations and Special Occasions 83

Chapter 8: Lifestyle Changes for Managing Acid Reflux 87

Tips for Improving Digestion and Reducing Stress 87

Incorporating Exercise into Your Routine 91
Getting Quality Sleep to Prevent Acid Reflux Episodes 94
30 DAYS MEAL PLAN 96
Conclusion.. 98

Introduction

Once upon a time, in a bustling metropolis full of many cultures and cuisines, there lived a woman named Emily who suffered from a common but terrible condition: acid reflux. Despite her passion of eating new dishes and experimenting in the kitchen, Emily's illness hindered her ability to do so, since she was always battling symptoms such as heartburn and indigestion. Emily came upon "The Acid Reflux Cookbook" while visiting her favorite bookstore.

She grabbed it up and started flicking through the pages, intrigued. To her amazement, she discovered a treasure mine of delectable dishes that are mild on the digestive system and help to relieve acid reflux symptoms. From substantial breakfasts to fulfilling dinners and even delicious desserts, the cookbook provided a diverse selection of tempting foods produced with healthful ingredients and customized to the requirements of acid reflux sufferers. Each dish was carefully developed to be both delectable and easy on the stomach, allowing Emily to eat her favorite meals without concern of discomfort.

But the book included more than simply recipes. It also offered significant insights on diet-based acid reflux management, including tips on detecting trigger foods, planning meals for optimal digestion, and making better restaurant choices. Emily felt empowered as she learned how to confidently handle social situations and special events, equipped with the knowledge and tools to enjoy food without restriction.

As Emily went through the pages of "The Acid Reflux Cookbook," she realized it was more than simply a compilation of recipes; it was a road map to greater health and fitness. Emily was inspired by the book's practical counsel, tasty recipes, and emotional encouragement to begin on a path toward a happier, healthier life free of the confines of acid reflux. Emily was filled with excitement and expectation, knowing she had discovered a reliable friend on her quest for gastronomic independence. With "The Acid Reflux Cookbook" at her side, she eagerly anticipated relishing every moment, meal, and bite, knowing that she was feeding her body and spirit with food that not only tasted good but also made her feel wonderful.

So, with a grin on her face and a spring in her step, Emily bought the book and began a new chapter in her culinary adventures. With each recipe she attempted and every meal she ate, she felt grateful for the gift of excellent health and the delight of wonderful cuisine, knowing she had discovered her ultimate guide to living well with acid reflux.

Chapter 1: Understanding Acid Reflux

What is Acid Reflux?

Acid reflux is a frequent medical disorder in which stomach acid rushes back into the esophagus, producing irritation and pain. Acid reflux, also known as gastroesophageal reflux disease (GERD), has a range of symptoms from moderate to severe.

The digestive system is a complicated network of organs that breaks down food and absorbs nutrients. When we eat, food goes down the esophagus and into the stomach, where it is digested by gastric acid. Normally, a muscular valve known as the lower esophageal sphincter (LES) stops stomach acid from refluxing into the esophagus by shutting strongly after food passes. However, in situations of acid reflux, the LES may become weaker or relax abnormally, enabling stomach acid to flow backward.

Several factors can contribute to the development of acid reflux. These include:

1. **Diet:** Spicy, fatty, or acidic meals, coffee, alcohol, and carbonated drinks can worsen acid reflux symptoms.

2. **Lifestyle habits:** Smoking, excessive alcohol use, and obesity can trigger acid reflux by disrupting LES function and increasing stomach acid production.
3. **Medical conditions:** Hiatal hernia, gastroparesis, and peptic ulcers can interrupt digestion and cause acid reflux.
4. Certain medicines, such as NSAIDs, calcium channel blockers, and asthma treatments, might increase the risk of acid reflux as a side effect.

If left untreated, acid reflux can cause consequences such as esophagitis (esophageal inflammation), esophageal strictures (esophageal constriction), Barrett's oesophagus (a precancerous disease), and, in rare situations, esophageal cancer.

Acid reflux is normally diagnosed using a medical history, physical examination, and diagnostic testing such endoscopy, pH monitoring, and esophageal manometry. Acid reflux treatment options include lifestyle adjustments, dietary changes, drugs to lower stomach acid production, and, in severe instances, surgery to repair or strengthen the LES.

Understanding the underlying causes and processes of acid reflux is critical for managing and preventing symptoms. Individuals can reduce discomfort and enhance quality of life by taking a comprehensive approach to therapy and implementing acid reflux-friendly behaviours into their everyday lives.

Causes and Triggers of Acid Reflux

Acid reflux is a frequent digestive condition defined by the backward passage of stomach acid into the oesophagus. While occasional bouts of acid reflux are natural and may not cause substantial pain, persistent or regular occurrences can lead to issues and impair general health.

Recognising the origins and triggers of acid reflux is an important part of comprehending the condition. Acid reflux can be caused by a variety of causes, including lifestyle behaviours and underlying medical issues.

One of the most common causes of acid reflux is a weak or malfunctioning lower esophageal sphincter (LES). The LES is a ring of muscle at the bottom of the oesophagus that serves as a barrier between the oesophagus and the stomach. When it works properly, the LES opens to

In addition to structural abnormalities, certain lifestyle habits and dietary factors can trigger or exacerbate acid reflux symptoms. These may include:

1. Eating large meals or lying down immediately after eating
2. Consuming spicy, acidic, or fatty foods
3. Drinking alcohol or caffeinated beverages

4. Smoking or using tobacco products
5. Being overweight or obese
6. Wearing tight clothing that puts pressure on the abdomen 7. Stress and anxiety

Furthermore, several medical problems and drugs might exacerbate acid reflux symptoms. Conditions such as gastroesophageal reflux disease (GERD), gastroparesis, and peptic ulcers can all increase the incidence of acid reflux. Similarly, medicines such nonsteroidal anti-inflammatory drugs (NSAIDs), calcium channel blockers, and certain antidepressants can relax the LES or irritate the oesophagus, causing acid reflux symptoms. Overall, knowing the origins and triggers of acid reflux is critical for successfully managing the illness and lowering the frequency and severity of symptoms. Individuals with acid reflux can improve their quality of life by recognising and avoiding potential triggers, adopting lifestyle changes, and obtaining appropriate medical treatment.

Symptoms of Acid Reflux

Acid reflux, commonly known as gastroesophageal reflux disease (GERD), is a common digestive ailment in which stomach acid backs up into the oesophagus. This acid backflow can induce a wide range of symptoms, from minor to severe, and can have a substantial influence on a person's quality of life. One of the most prevalent acid reflux symptoms is heartburn, which is a burning sensation in the chest that usually comes after eating or lying down. This sensation may intensify while bending over or resting flat, and it is sometimes mistaken for a heart attack due to its severity. Regurgitation is another acid reflux symptom that causes stomach contents to come back up into the throat or mouth. This can cause a sour or bitter taste in the mouth, as well as the sensation of food or liquid rising back up into the throat. Many people with acid reflux have trouble swallowing, a condition known as dysphagia. This can range from feeling like food is trapped in your throat to pain or discomfort during swallowing, which may be accompanied by chest or throat stiffness.

In addition to these primary symptoms, acid reflux can also manifest in other ways, such as:

1. Chronic coughing or hoarseness, often due to irritation of the throat by stomach acid.

2. Sore throat or throat clearing, which may be persistent and accompanied by a raspy voice.
3. Asthma-like symptoms, including wheezing or difficulty breathing, especially when lying down.
4. Dental erosion or tooth decay, as a result of repeated exposure to stomach acid.
5. Nausea or vomiting, particularly after meals or when lying down.

It's important to note that the severity and frequency of acid reflux symptoms can vary from person to person, and some individuals may experience occasional mild symptoms while others may have chronic and debilitating symptoms that require medical intervention.

Overall, recognizing the symptoms of acid reflux is the first step towards effectively managing the condition and improving quality of life. By understanding the signs of acid reflux and seeking appropriate treatment, individuals can take control of their digestive health and find relief from the discomfort and disruption caused by this common ailment.

Complications of Untreated Acid Reflux

Understanding the dangers of untreated acid reflux is critical for everyone who has symptoms of the illness. Acid reflux occurs when the stomach's acidic contents flow back into the oesophagus, producing irritation and pain. While brief bouts of acid reflux are normal and usually innocuous, persistent or untreated acid reflux can result in significant consequences over time.

Esophagitis, or inflammation of the oesophagus, is one of the most prevalent consequences of untreated acid reflux disease. When stomach acid regularly contacts the esophageal lining, it can cause irritation, edoema, and tissue damage. This can cause symptoms such as chest discomfort, trouble swallowing, and the sensation of food stuck in the throat.

In extreme situations, untreated esophagitis can result in problems such as esophageal ulcers or strictures. Esophageal ulcers are open sores on the esophageal lining, whereas strictures are narrowings caused by scar tissue development. Both of these disorders can cause difficulties swallowing and may need medical intervention to address.

Barrett's oesophagus is another potential consequence of untreated acid reflux. This is a disorder in which the cells lining the oesophagus alter as a result of continuous stomach acid exposure. Barrett's oesophagus is considered a precancerous disease since it raises the likelihood of developing esophageal cancer over time. Regular monitoring and care of Barrett's oesophagus are critical for lowering the risk of cancer development.

In addition to esophageal issues, untreated acid reflux can harm other sections of the digestive system. Chronic inflammation of the throat and vocal chords can result in laryngitis or chronic cough. Tooth erosion and cavities are two dental disorders that can arise when tooth enamel is exposed to stomach acid.

Furthermore, untreated acid reflux can impair general quality of life, including sleep disruptions, decreased productivity, and emotional anguish. Persistent acid reflux sensations can lead to anxiety and stress, increasing the cycle of discomfort and worsening symptoms.

Overall, the implications of untreated acid reflux highlight the necessity of early detection and appropriate treatment of the problem. Individuals can lower the risk of problems and enhance their general health and well-being by making essential lifestyle adjustments, dietary alterations, and medical treatments. The Acid

Reflux Cookbook strives to give practical advice and tasty dishes to help people manage acid reflux symptoms and avoid problems, resulting in a better and happier life.

Chapter 2: Managing Acid Reflux Through Diet

The Role of Diet in Acid Reflux Management

Understanding the significance of nutrition in acid reflux management is critical for anybody seeking relief from this painful illness. Acid reflux occurs when stomach acid runs back into the oesophagus, resulting in symptoms including heartburn, regurgitation, and chest discomfort. While many factors can contribute to acid reflux, including lifestyle behaviours and underlying medical disorders, nutrition plays an important role in both triggering and treating symptoms.

Certain foods and beverages have been shown to increase acid reflux symptoms and should be avoided or consumed in moderation. These include spicy meals, acidic fruits, citrus juices, fatty or fried foods, carbonated beverages, caffeine, and alcohol. Large meals and late-night dining, as well as lying down shortly after eating, can all increase the risk of suffering acid reflux symptoms.

On the other hand, there are foods and dietary habits that may help alleviate symptoms of acid reflux and promote digestive health. These include:

Consuming fiber-rich meals such as fruits, vegetables, whole grains, and legumes helps improve digestion and avoid constipation.

Choose lean proteins, including poultry, fish, tofu, and beans, over fatty or fried meats, which can be difficult to digest and cause acid reflux.

Choose low-acid fruits and vegetables, such bananas, melons, apples, carrots, and green leafy vegetables, to reduce acid reflux symptoms.

Consuming probiotic-rich foods like yoghurt, kefir, sauerkraut, and kombucha can promote gut health and decrease inflammation in the digestive tract.

Stay hydrated and help digestion by drinking lots of water throughout the day. Limit consumption of fizzy and caffeinated beverages.

Individuals suffering with acid reflux can effectively control their symptoms and enhance their overall quality of life by making wise food choices and establishing healthy eating habits.

The Acid Reflux Cookbook has a plethora of tasty recipes and practical guidance for incorporating acid reflux-friendly foods into your daily routine, allowing you to eat fulfilling meals without worry of discomfort. With its help, you may regain control of your diet and alleviate acid reflux problems one delicious meal at a time.

Foods to Avoid for Acid Reflux

When controlling acid reflux via nutrition, it is critical to be aware of the items that might increase symptoms and cause discomfort. Individuals with acid reflux who understand which foods to avoid can take proactive actions to reduce their likelihood of suffering heartburn, regurgitation, and other unpleasant symptoms. High-fat meals are one type of food to avoid if you have acid reflux since they delay stomach emptying and increase the probability of reflux. High-fat foods include fried dishes, fatty meats, full-fat dairy items, and decadent sweets. These products can relax the lower esophageal sphincter (LES), enabling stomach acid to flow back up into the oesophagus.

Spicy meals can also irritate the esophageal lining, causing acid reflux symptoms. Common spicy foods to avoid include hot peppers, chilli peppers, salsa, and spicy sauces. For people who suffer from acid reflux, using milder seasonings might help alleviate the symptoms.

Acidic meals and beverages have also been linked to increased acid reflux symptoms. Citrus fruits and juices (oranges, lemons, and grapefruits), tomatoes and tomato-based goods (marinara sauce and ketchup), and carbonated and caffeinated beverages (coffee, tea, and soda) are all examples. These acidic chemicals might irritate the oesophagus and worsen acid reflux symptoms. Additionally, carbonated and alcoholic beverages can weaken the LES and increase stomach acid production, therefore they should be avoided by people who have acid reflux. Alcohol, in particular, relaxes the LES and impairs esophageal function, increasing the incidence of reflux episodes.

Finally, people with acid reflux should minimise their consumption of chocolate and peppermint, since these foods might relax the LES and exacerbate reflux symptoms. While chocolate and peppermint are popular sweets, individuals who suffer from acid reflux should consume them in moderation or avoid them completely.

Individuals with acid reflux can enhance their quality of life by being aware of these common trigger foods and making intelligent dietary choices. While some changes and experimentation may be required, the benefits of reduced discomfort and improved digestive health can make the effort worthwhile.

Foods that May Help Alleviate Acid Reflux Symptoms

Dietary changes are essential for relieving acid reflux symptoms. Making wise dietary choices can help to lessen the frequency and severity of reflux episodes. In this chapter, we'll look at the different foods that can help relieve acid reflux symptoms, as well as how to include them into your meals using the Acid Reflux Cookbook.

Non-citrus fruits are one type of meal that may help relieve acid reflux symptoms. While citrus fruits like oranges and lemons have been known to cause reflux in some people, fruits like bananas, melons, and apples are usually thought to be softer on the digestive system. These fruits are not only tasty, but they also contain vital vitamins, minerals, and fibre that promote digestive health.

Similarly, some veggies can help reduce acid reflux symptoms. Leafy greens like spinach and kale, as well as non-starchy veggies like broccoli, cauliflower, and cucumbers, are ideal for people suffering with acid reflux. These veggies are low in acidity and high in nutrients, making them excellent for use in acid refluxfriendly meals.

Whole grains are another type of food that may help relieve acid reflux symptoms. Whole grains such as oats, brown rice, quinoa, and barley can help those with acid reflux. These grains are strong in fibre and complex carbs, which can help you feel full and improve your digestive health.

In addition to fruits, vegetables, and healthy grains, lean proteins can help manage acid reflux. Foods like skinless fowl, fish, tofu, and lentils are high in protein and less prone to cause reflux symptoms than fatty or fried meats. By integrating lean proteins into your meals, you may aid in muscle repair and maintenance while avoiding acid reflux.

Finally, when taken in moderation, several herbs and spices can help relieve acid reflux symptoms. Ginger, for example, has been used for generations as a natural treatment for indigestion and nausea. Similarly, herbs such as parsley, basil, and cilantro can enhance the flavour of foods while preventing reflux symptoms.

Incorporating these items into your diet will help reduce acid reflux symptoms and improve overall digestive health. The Acid Reflux Cookbook provides information and tasty dishes to help you enjoy a diverse and enjoyable diet while properly controlling acid reflux symptoms. Making careful food choices allows you to take charge of your health and well-being one meal at a time.

Tips for Eating and Drinking to Prevent Acid Reflux

When controlling acid reflux through nutrition, it is critical to develop healthy eating and drinking habits that can help relieve symptoms and avoid discomfort. You may effectively control acid reflux and improve your quality of life by making thoughtful decisions and paying attention to how and what you eat.

First and foremost, limit your portion sizes and prevent overeating, since excess food consumption can put pressure on the stomach and increase the chance of acid reflux attacks. Eat smaller, more frequent meals throughout the day, rather than large, heavy meals, which can exacerbate symptoms.

Also, pay attention to the timing of your meals and avoid eating late at night or straight before bed. Lying down after eating might worsen acid reflux symptoms, so leave as least two to three hours between your previous meal and bedtime.

When selecting meals, choose lean proteins like poultry, fish, and tofu, which are simpler to digest and less prone to cause acid reflux. Consume plenty of fruits and vegetables, as they provide critical nutrients and fibre while being naturally low in fat and acid.

Consuming high-fat and spicy foods might irritate the oesophagus and worsen acid reflux symptoms. Instead, use low-fat cooking methods like baking, grilling, or steaming, and season your food with herbs and spices rather than heavy sauces or condiments.

In addition to dietary choices, be mindful of what you drink, since some beverages might aggravate acid reflux symptoms. Avoid carbonated drinks, caffeinated beverages, and alcohol since they relax the lower esophageal sphincter and increase the risk of acid reflux.

Instead, drink water, herbal teas, and non-acidic fruit juices to keep hydrated and ease your digestive tract.

Finally, listen to your body and observe how various meals and beverages impact your symptoms. Keep a food journal to track your consumption and identify potential triggers, and consider speaking with a healthcare practitioner or certified dietitian for further personalised advice and assistance.

You may take charge of your diet and successfully manage your symptoms by following these acid reflux-prevention eating and drinking suggestions. With the Acid Reflux Cookbook, you'll have access to tasty and healthy dishes that are easy on your digestive system, allowing you to eat without concern of discomfort or disturbance.

Chapter 3: Meal Planning for Acid Reflux

Principles of Acid Reflux-Friendly Meal Planning

In "The Acid Reflux Cookbook," Chapter 3 dives into the fundamentals of acid reflux-friendly meal planning, offering readers with a complete approach to designing balanced and calming meals that support digestive health and ease acid reflux symptoms.

Meal planning for acid reflux begins with choosing meals that are mild on the digestive tract and reduce the likelihood of triggering reflux episodes. This entails prioritising nutrient-dense whole meals while avoiding those that are known to aggravate symptoms, such as spicy, acidic, fatty, and caffeine.

One major tenet of acid reflux-friendly meal planning is to focus on lean proteins like poultry, fish, tofu, and lentils, which supply necessary nutrients without adding extra fat or acidity to the diet. These protein sources improve satiety and muscle maintenance and repair while minimising intestinal stress.

Acid reflux-friendly meals should contain a variety of non-starchy vegetables, such as leafy greens, broccoli, cauliflower, and bell peppers, which are high in vitamins, minerals, and fibre. These veggies aid digestion, maintain gut health, and add a delicious crunch and texture to meals without causing reflux symptoms.

Whole grains and complex carbs are also crucial components of acid reflux-friendly meal planning, since they provide long-lasting energy and fibre to aid digestion and encourage feelings of fullness. Choose whole grain choices such as brown rice, quinoa, oats, and whole wheat bread, which are less likely to cause reflux than refined grains.

When preparing meals for acid reflux, consider food quantities and meal scheduling. Eating smaller, more frequent meals throughout the day can help to minimise overeating and lower the likelihood of reflux symptoms, while also allowing the digestive system to work more effectively. Avoiding heavy meals, particularly before bedtime, can also assist to reduce nocturnal reflux symptoms.

Finally, consuming healthy fats in moderation might benefit acid reflux patients since certain fats, such as those found in avocados, nuts, seeds, and olive oil, have anti-inflammatory characteristics and may aid to relax the digestive system. However, it is critical to limit your intake of high-fat meals, fried foods, and thick sauces, which can increase reflux symptoms.

By following these acid reflux-friendly meal planning guidelines, readers of "The Acid Reflux Cookbook" may prepare tasty and gratifying meals that improve digestive health and general wellbeing. With a focus on complete, nutrient-dense foods and mindful eating practices, meal planning for acid reflux becomes a straightforward and fun process, allowing readers to regain control of their diet and lessen acid reflux symptoms.

Sample Meal Plans for Breakfast, Lunch, and Dinner

Chapter 3 of the Acid Reflux Cookbook has a plethora of meal planning options that are particularly designed to treat acid reflux symptoms. These sample meal plans for breakfast, lunch, and supper are intended to be mild on the digestive system while yet giving delicious and filling alternatives throughout the day.

Start your day with a full but calming breakfast that will not irritate acid reflux symptoms. Consider starting your day with a bowl of muesli topped with sliced bananas and almonds for extra texture and flavour.

Muesli is an excellent choice for persons with acid reflux since it is low in acidity and high in fibre, which can help to regulate digestion and alleviate symptoms. For a refreshing start to the day, try pairing your muesli with a cup of herbal tea or a glass of non-acidic fruit juice.

When it comes to lunch, choose light and nutritious selections that will not weigh you down or cause acid reflux symptoms. Quinoa salad with grilled chicken is a delicious and easy-to-digest noon meal.

Quinoa is a gluten-free grain that is easy on the digestive system and high in protein and fibre, making it an excellent choice for those with acid reflux. Load your salad with fresh veggies like leafy greens, cucumbers, and cherry tomatoes, then drizzle with a tangy vinaigrette prepared with olive oil and lemon juice for more flavour.

For dinner, choose for simple yet soothing foods that will help to alleviate any remaining acid reflux symptoms and encourage peaceful sleep.

Baked chicken breast is lean and simple to digest, while roasted veggies such as carrots, broccoli, and bell peppers are high in vitamins and minerals that promote digestive health. Serve your chicken and veggies with a small serving of brown rice or quinoa for extra fibre and satiety.

With these sample meal plans for breakfast, lunch, and supper, you may eat tasty and fulfilling meals while managing your acid reflux. You may alleviate discomfort and live a more vibrant and full life by eating soft and nutritious foods that promote digestive health.

Snack Ideas for Acid Reflux Relief

Finding appropriate snacks that provide symptom relief can be critical when managing acid reflux through diet. Snacks help to keep blood sugar levels stable throughout the day and can prevent overeating during main meals. The Acid Reflux Cookbook contains a variety of snack ideas that are both delicious and satisfying while also relieving acid reflux symptoms.

Greek yoghurt with honey and almonds is a tasty and light snack option. Greek yoghurt is high in protein and probiotics, which can promote digestive health and reduce inflammation. A drizzle of honey adds sweetness without overwhelming the stomach, while almonds add healthy fats and crunch.

Another snack option is almond butter and banana rice cakes. Almond butter is a nutritious spread that contains heart-healthy fats and protein, making it a filling option for keeping hunger at bay. Spread it on rice cakes for a gluten-free and digestible base, then top with banana slices for extra flavour and potassium.

For those looking for something refreshing and hydrating, a cucumber and hummus snack platter is an excellent option. Cucumbers have low acidity and a high water content, making them gentle on the stomach and hydrating. Pair them with a creamy and flavorful hummus dip for a nutritious snack that's easy on the stomach.

In addition to these options, The Acid Reflux Cookbook offers suggestions for making balanced and acid reflux-friendly snacks with common household ingredients. By focusing on whole foods, avoiding trigger ingredients, and eating small, frequent meals throughout the day, you can help relieve acid reflux symptoms while still enjoying delicious and nourishing snacks.

Whether you're looking for a quick bite between meals or a satisfying treat to satisfy your cravings, The Acid Reflux Cookbook's snack ideas cater to a wide range of tastes and dietary requirements. With these snacks at your disposal, you can snack with confidence knowing that you're improving your digestive health and effectively managing acid reflux.

Chapter 4: Acid Reflux Friendly Recipes

Breakfast Recipes

Oatmeal with Bananas and Almonds

Ingredients:

1. 1/2 cup old-fashioned rolled oats
2. 1 cup water or milk (dairy or plant-based)
3. 1 ripe banana, sliced
4. 2 tablespoons sliced almonds
5. 1 teaspoon honey (optional)
6. Pinch of cinnamon (optional)

Instructions:

1. In a small saucepan, bring the water or milk to a boil over medium heat.
2. Stir in the rolled oats and reduce the heat to low. Simmer for 57 minutes, stirring occasionally, until the oats are thick and creamy.
3. Remove the saucepan from the heat and let the oatmeal cool slightly.

4. Transfer the oatmeal to a serving bowl and top with sliced bananas and almonds.

5. Drizzle with honey and sprinkle with cinnamon, if desired.

6. Serve warm and enjoy

Nutritional Information (per serving):

1. Calories: 300
2. Fat: 9g
3. Protein: 7g
4. Carbohydrates: 51g
5. Fiber: 8g
6. Sugars: 15g

Serving Size: 1 bowl

Cooking Time: 10 minutes

Greek Yogurt Parfait with Berries

Ingredients:

1. 1 cup plain Greek yogurt
2. ½ cup mixed berries (such as strawberries, blueberries, and raspberries)
3. 2 tbsp honey or maple syrup (optional)
4. ¼ cup granola (optional)
5. Fresh mint leaves for garnish (optional)

Instructions:

1. In a small bowl, layer the Greek yogurt with the mixed berries.
2. If desired, drizzle honey or maple syrup over the yogurt and berries for added sweetness.
3. Top the parfait with granola for extra crunch and texture.
4. Garnish with fresh mint leaves for a pop of color and flavor.
5. Serve immediately and enjoy!

Nutritional Information (per serving):

1. Calories: 200
2. Fat: 4g

3. Protein: 18g
4. Carbohydrates: 25g
5. Fiber: 3g
6. Sugars: 18g

Serving Size: 1 serving

Cooking Time: 5 minutes

Egg White Veggie Omelet

Ingredients:

1. 4 egg whites
2. 1/4 cup diced bell peppers (any color)
3. 1/4 cup diced onions
4. 1/4 cup diced tomatoes
5. 1/4 cup chopped spinach
6. 1/4 cup sliced mushrooms
7. 1 teaspoon olive oil
8. Salt and pepper to taste

Instructions:

1. Heat olive oil in a non-stick skillet over medium heat.
2. Add diced onions and bell peppers to the skillet and sauté until softened, about 2-3 minutes.
3. Add mushrooms and cook for another 2 minutes until they start to brown.
4. Stir in diced tomatoes and chopped spinach, and cook for an additional 1-2 minutes until spinach is wilted.
5. In a separate bowl, whisk the egg whites until frothy.

6. Pour the whisked egg whites over the vegetable mixture in the skillet.

7. Allow the omelet to cook undisturbed for about 2-3 minutes, or until the edges start to set.

8. Using a spatula, gently lift the edges of the omelet and tilt the skillet to allow any uncooked egg to flow underneath.

9. Once the omelet is mostly set, carefully flip it over and cook for another 1-2 minutes, or until cooked through.

10. Season with salt and pepper to taste.

11. Slide the omelet onto a plate and serve hot.

Nutritional Information (per serving):

1. Calories: 80
2. Protein: 14g
3. Carbohydrates: 4g
4. Fat: 2g
5. Fiber: 1g
6. Sugar: 2g
7. Sodium: 270mg

Serving Size:

- This recipe makes one serving.

Cooking Time:

- Approximately 10 minutes.

Lunch Recipes

Quinoa Salad with Grilled Chicken

Ingredients:

1. 1 cup quinoa
2. 2 cups water or low-sodium chicken broth
3. 1 pound boneless, skinless chicken breasts
4. 1 tablespoon olive oil
5. Salt and pepper to taste
6. 1 red bell pepper, diced
7. 1 cucumber, diced
8. 1/4 cup red onion, finely chopped
9. 1/4 cup fresh parsley, chopped
10. 2 tablespoons lemon juice
11. 2 tablespoons extra virgin olive oil
12. 1 clove garlic, minced
13. Optional: 1/4 cup crumbled feta cheese (for non-vegan option)

Instructions:

1. Rinse the quinoa under cold water using a fine mesh strainer. In a medium saucepan, combine quinoa and water or chicken broth. Bring to a boil, then reduce heat to low, cover, and simmer for 1520

minutes, or until quinoa is cooked and liquid is absorbed. Remove from heat and let it cool.

2. Preheat grill or grill pan over medium-high heat. Brush chicken breasts with olive oil and season with salt and pepper. Grill chicken for 6-7 minutes on each side, or until cooked through and no longer pink in the center. Remove from grill and let it rest for a few minutes before slicing.

3. In a large mixing bowl, combine cooked quinoa, diced bell pepper, cucumber, red onion, and parsley.

4. In a small bowl, whisk together lemon juice, extra virgin olive oil, and minced garlic to make the dressing.

5. Add sliced grilled chicken to the quinoa salad mixture. Pour the dressing over the salad and toss until well combined. If using, sprinkle crumbled feta cheese on top.

6. Serve immediately or refrigerate for later. Enjoy!

Nutritional Information:

1. Serving Size: 1/4 of recipe
2. Calories: 350
3. Total Fat: 15g
4. Saturated Fat: 3g
5. Cholesterol: 75mg

6. Sodium: 250mg
7. Total Carbohydrates: 28g
8. Dietary Fiber: 4g
9. Sugars: 3g
10. Protein: 26g

Cooking Time:

1. Preparation: 10 minutes
2. Cooking: 20 minutes
3. Total Time: 30 minutes

Turkey and Avocado Wrap

Ingredients:

1. 4 large whole wheat or spinach tortillas
2. 1 lb sliced turkey breast
3. 2 ripe avocados, sliced
4. 1 cup shredded lettuce
5. 1 large tomato, sliced
6. 1/4 cup thinly sliced red onion
7. 1/4 cup chopped fresh cilantro
8. 1/4 cup plain Greek yogurt (optional)
9. Salt and pepper to taste

Instructions:

1. Lay out the tortillas on a clean surface.
2. Evenly distribute the turkey slices onto each tortilla.
3. Layer the sliced avocado, lettuce, tomato, red onion, and cilantro on top of the turkey.
4. If desired, spread a thin layer of Greek yogurt over the ingredients.
5. Season with salt and pepper to taste.

6. Roll up the tortillas tightly, tucking in the sides as you go, to form wraps.

7. Cut each wrap in half diagonally for easier handling.

Nutritional Information (per serving):

1. Calories: 350
2. Total Fat: 14g
3. Saturated Fat: 3g
4. Cholesterol: 60mg
5. Sodium: 700mg
6. Total Carbohydrates: 35g
7. Dietary Fiber: 8g
8. Sugars: 4g
9. Protein: 25g

Serving Size: 1 wrap

Cooking Time: 15 minutes

Salmon and Vegetable Stir-Fry

Ingredients:

1. 1 pound of fresh salmon fillets, skin removed and cut into cubes
2. 2 cups of mixed vegetables (such as bell peppers, broccoli, carrots, and snap peas), chopped
3. 2 cloves of garlic, minced
4. 1 tablespoon of ginger, minced
5. 2 tablespoons of low-sodium soy sauce
6. 1 tablespoon of sesame oil
7. 1 tablespoon of olive oil
8. 1 tablespoon of honey
9. Salt and pepper to taste
10. Optional: cooked brown rice or quinoa for serving

Instructions:

1. In a small bowl, mix together the soy sauce, sesame oil, olive oil, honey, garlic, and ginger to make the marinade.

2. Place the cubed salmon in a shallow dish and pour the marinade over it, ensuring each piece is coated evenly. Let it marinate for about 15-20 minutes in the refrigerator.

3. Heat a large skillet or wok over medium-high heat. Once hot, add the marinated salmon cubes (reserving the marinade) and cook for 2-3 minutes on each side until lightly browned and cooked through. Remove the salmon from the skillet and set aside.

4. In the same skillet, add the chopped vegetables and stir-fry for 3-4 minutes until they are tender yet crisp.

5. Pour the reserved marinade into the skillet with the vegetables and stir well, allowing it to thicken slightly.

6. Return the cooked salmon to the skillet and toss everything together gently, ensuring the salmon and vegetables are coated in the sauce.

7. Season with salt and pepper to taste.

8. Serve the salmon and vegetable stir-fry hot, optionally over cooked brown rice or quinoa.

Nutritional Information (per serving, without rice/quinoa):

1. Calories: 280
2. Total Fat: 15g

3. Saturated Fat: 2.5g
4. Cholesterol: 70mg
5. Sodium: 400mg
6. Total Carbohydrates: 10g
7. Dietary Fiber: 2g
8. Sugars: 6g
9. Protein: 26g

Serving Size: This recipe makes 4 servings.

Cooking Time: Approximately 25 minutes, including preparation and cooking time.

Dinner Recipes

Baked Chicken Breast with Roasted Vegetables

Ingredients:

1. 4 boneless, skinless chicken breasts
2. 2 cups mixed vegetables (such as bell peppers, zucchini, and carrots), chopped
3. 2 tablespoons olive oil
4. 1 teaspoon dried thyme
5. 1 teaspoon dried rosemary
6. 1 teaspoon garlic powder
7. Salt and pepper to taste

Instructions:

1. Preheat your oven to 400°F (200°C).
2. Place the chicken breasts in a baking dish and season them with thyme, rosemary, garlic powder, salt, and pepper.
3. In a separate bowl, toss the mixed vegetables with olive oil, salt, and pepper until evenly coated.

4. Arrange the seasoned vegetables around the chicken breasts in the baking dish.
5. Cover the baking dish with aluminum foil and bake in the preheated oven for 25-30 minutes, or until the chicken is cooked through and reaches an internal temperature of 165°F (74°C).
6. Remove the foil during the last 10 minutes of baking to allow the chicken and vegetables to brown slightly.
7. Once cooked, remove the baking dish from the oven and let it rest for a few minutes before serving.

Nutritional Information (per serving):

1. Calories: 250
2. Total Fat: 10g
3. Saturated Fat: 2g
4. Cholesterol: 100mg
5. Sodium: 200mg
6. Total Carbohydrates: 6g
7. Dietary Fiber: 2g
8. Sugars: 2g
9. Protein: 35g

Serving Size: 1 chicken breast with vegetables

Cooking Time: 25-30 minutes

Shrimp and Vegetable Skewers

Ingredients:

1. 1 pound large shrimp, peeled and deveined
2. 1 zucchini, sliced into rounds
3. 1 yellow bell pepper, cut into chunks
4. 1 red onion, cut into chunks
5. 8 cherry tomatoes
6. 2 tablespoons olive oil
7. 2 cloves garlic, minced
8. 1 teaspoon dried oregano
9. 1 teaspoon dried basil
10. Salt and pepper to taste
11. Wooden skewers, soaked in water for 30 minutes

Instructions:

1. Preheat your grill to medium-high heat.
2. In a small bowl, mix together olive oil, minced garlic, oregano, basil, salt, and pepper.
3. Thread shrimp, zucchini, bell pepper, onion, and cherry tomatoes onto the soaked wooden skewers, alternating between ingredients.

4. Brush the skewers with the prepared olive oil mixture, coating them evenly.
5. Place the skewers on the preheated grill and cook for 2-3 minutes per side, or until the shrimp are pink and opaque and the vegetables are tender and slightly charred.
6. Once cooked, remove the skewers from the grill and let them rest for a few minutes before serving.
7. Serve the shrimp and vegetable skewers hot, optionally with a side of rice or a green salad.

Nutritional Information:

1. Serving Size: 1 skewer
2. Calories: 160
3. Total Fat: 7g
4. Saturated Fat: 1g
5. Cholesterol: 143mg
6. Sodium: 290mg
7. Total Carbohydrates: 8g
8. Dietary Fiber: 2g
9. Sugars: 4g
10. Protein: 17g

Cooking Time: 10-15 minutes

Vegetable and Lentil Soup

Vegetable and lentil soup is a tasty and soothing dish that is not only simple to cook but also mild on the stomach, making it an ideal choice for individuals suffering from acid reflux. This dish, packed with healthful foods and delicious herbs, is an excellent addition to any acid reflux cookbook.

Below are extensive directions for preparing this recipe, as well as nutritional information, serving size, and cooking time.

Ingredients:

1. 1 tablespoon olive oil
2. 1 medium onion, diced
3. 2 cloves garlic, minced
4. 2 medium carrots, diced
5. 2 celery stalks, diced
6. 1 cup dried lentils, rinsed
7. 4 cups low-sodium vegetable broth
8. 1 can (14.5 ounces) diced tomatoes, undrained
9. 1 teaspoon dried thyme
10. 1 teaspoon dried oregano
11. Salt and pepper to taste

12. Fresh parsley for garnish (optional)

Instructions:

1. In a large pot, heat the olive oil over medium heat. Add the diced onion and cook until softened, about 5 minutes.

2. Add the minced garlic to the pot and cook for an additional 1-2 minutes, until fragrant.

3. Add the diced carrots and celery to the pot and cook for another 5 minutes, stirring occasionally.

4. Stir in the rinsed lentils, vegetable broth, diced tomatoes (with their juices), dried thyme, and dried oregano. Bring the mixture to a boil.

5. Once boiling, reduce the heat to low, cover the pot, and let the soup simmer for about 20-25 minutes, or until the lentils and vegetables are tender.

6. Season the soup with salt and pepper to taste. Adjust the seasoning as needed.

7. Serve the soup hot, garnished with fresh parsley if desired.

Nutritional Information (per serving):

1. Calories: 220
2. Total Fat: 4g
3. Saturated Fat: 0.5g
4. Cholesterol: 0mg
5. Sodium: 480mg
6. Total Carbohydrates: 36g
7. Dietary Fiber: 14g
8. Sugars: 6g
9. Protein: 12g

Serving Size: This recipe makes approximately 4 servings.

Cooking Time: Approximately 40 minutes from start to finish.

Snack Recipes

Almond Butter and Banana Rice Cakes

Ingredients:

1. 4 rice cakes (preferably whole grain)
2. ½ cup almond butter
3. 2 ripe bananas, thinly sliced
4. Honey or maple syrup (optional, for drizzling)
5. Cinnamon powder (optional, for sprinkling)

Instructions:

1. Spread a generous layer of almond butter evenly on each rice cake.
2. Place thinly sliced bananas on top of the almond butter layer.
3. Optionally, drizzle honey or maple syrup over the banana slices for added sweetness.
4. Sprinkle cinnamon powder lightly over the assembled rice cakes.
5. Serve immediately and enjoy!

Nutritional Information:

1. Serving Size: 1 rice cake with toppings
2. Calories: Approximately 180
3. Total Fat: 10g
4. Saturated Fat: 1g
5. Trans Fat: 0g
6. Cholesterol: 0mg
7. Sodium: 70mg
8. Total Carbohydrates: 20g
9. Dietary Fiber: 3g
10. Sugars: 7g
11. Protein: 5g

Cooking Time:

1. **Prep Time:** 5 minutes
2. **Cooking Time:** 0 minutes

Greek Yogurt with Honey and Almonds

Ingredients:

1. 1 cup Greek yogurt (plain, non-fat)
2. 1 tablespoon honey
3. 2 tablespoons sliced almonds

Instructions:

1. In a serving bowl, spoon out the Greek yogurt.
2. Drizzle the honey over the yogurt evenly.
3. Sprinkle the sliced almonds on top.

Nutritional Information:

1. Serving Size: 1 bowl (1 cup)
2. Calories: 220
3. Total Fat: 5g
4. Saturated Fat: 0.5g
5. Cholesterol: 10mg
6. Sodium: 50mg

7. Total Carbohydrates: 25g
8. Dietary Fiber: 2g
9. Sugars: 22g
10. Protein: 20g

Cooking Time: 5 minutes

Cucumber and Hummus Snack Platter

Ingredients:

1. 1 large cucumber
2. 1 cup of hummus (store-bought or homemade)

Instructions:

1. Wash the cucumber thoroughly under cold running water. Pat it dry with a clean kitchen towel.

2. Slice the cucumber into thin rounds or sticks, depending on your preference.

3. Arrange the cucumber slices or sticks on a serving platter.

4. Place the hummus in a small bowl in the center of the platter.

5. Serve immediately and enjoy!

Nutritional Information:

1. Cucumber: Cucumbers are low in calories and contain antioxidants, vitamins, and minerals such as vitamin K, potassium, and magnesium. They are also high in water content, making them hydrating and refreshing.

2. Hummus: Hummus is made primarily from chickpeas, which are a good source of plant-based protein and fiber. It also contains healthy fats from olive oil and tahini.

   Additionally, hummus provides essential nutrients such as iron, calcium, and vitamin C.

Serving Size: This recipe yields approximately 4 servings.

Cooking Time: There is no cooking required for this recipe, as it is a simple assembly of ingredients. It can be prepared in just a few minutes, making it a quick and convenient snack option.

Chapter 5: Beverages for Acid Reflux Relief

Herbal Teas for Soothing Acid Reflux

Herbal teas have long been known for their calming characteristics, making them a good alternative for anyone suffering from acid reflux symptoms.

These teas can help to soothe the digestive tract, decrease inflammation, and relieve acid reflux symptoms. Incorporating herbal teas into your daily routine might offer natural healing without the need of medicine. Here are some herbal teas that are very good for relieving acid reflux:

Chamomile Tea:

Chamomile is well-known for its soothing benefits on both the body and psyche.

It has anti-inflammatory qualities that can help relieve stomach discomfort and inflammation. Chamomile tea is also mild on the stomach, helping to relieve symptoms like heartburn and indigestion. Drinking chamomile tea after meals or before bedtime might help you relax and ease acid reflux symptoms.

Ginger Tea:

Ginger has been used for years as a natural treatment for a variety of digestive problems, including acid reflux. It includes chemicals that can neutralise stomach acid and aid digestion. Ginger tea is very good for alleviating nausea and pain caused by acid reflux. Simply soak fresh ginger slices or ginger tea bags in boiling water for a few minutes before straining and enjoying. Add honey or lemon for additional flavour and relaxing effects.

Licorice Root Tea:

Licorice root has been used in traditional medicine to alleviate gastrointestinal disorders, such as acid reflux. It includes chemicals that can coat and protect the esophageal lining, therefore minimising irritation and inflammation. Licorice root tea can also increase mucus production, which protects the stomach lining from excess acid. However, it is critical to use deglycyrrhizinated licorice (DGL) tea, as ordinary licorice root tea may have negative effects on blood pressure and potassium levels.

Peppermint Tea:

Peppermint is recognised for its cooling and calming effects, making it a popular remedy for intestinal distress. Peppermint tea can assist to calm the muscles of the digestive tract, lowering the risk of acid reflux. However, peppermint tea should be used with caution because it may exacerbate symptoms for some people. If peppermint tea worsens your acid reflux, stop drinking it and try another herbal tea.

Fennel Tea:

Fennel is a delicious plant that has been used for generations to assist digestion and relieve stomach discomfort. Fennel tea can help to relieve bloating, gas and indigestion, making it useful for people who have acid reflux. It includes chemicals that can relax digestive tract muscles and decrease inflammation. Drink a cup of fennel tea after meals to aid digestion and reduce acid reflux symptoms.

Incorporating herbal teas into your diet might help relieve acid reflux symptoms and improve overall digestive health. Experiment with several types of herbal teas to see which ones work best for you. Remember to check with your doctor before making any major changes to your diet or lifestyle, especially if you have underlying health issues or are on medicines.

Non-Acidic Fruit and Vegetable Juices

In the hunt for acid reflux treatment, non-acidic fruit and vegetable juices provide a delicious alternative. These beverages provide a tantalising variety of flavours without causing acid symptoms. Here, we look at a variety of non-acidic juices that may be easily incorporated into your acid reflux diet.

First, let's look at fruit juices that are mild on the stomach. One noteworthy choice is pear juice. Pear juice is known for its gentle flavour and low acidity, making it a calming drink that will not aggravate acid reflux problems. Similarly, apple juice prepared from low-acid apple cultivars can provide a delicious drink without creating pain.

Moving on to vegetable juices, cucumber juice stands out as a prominent candidate. Cucumber juice, with its high water content and neutral pH, replenishes the body while also soothing the digestive tract. Additionally, spinach juice is a good alternative.

Spinach juice is high in nutrients and has a moderate flavour, so it delivers a nutritious boost without causing acid reflux. Watermelon juice is another popular non-acidic choice. Watermelon juice is a pleasant beverage that is high in hydration and sweet. It can help relieve acid reflux symptoms. Its high water content improves digestion, making it an excellent addition to your acid reflux cookbook.

When making non-acidic fruit and vegetable juices, try combining different components to make delectable combinations. For example, combining cucumber, spinach, and pear may produce a delightful and calming beverage that helps digestive health. Experiment with different combinations to get the right balance of flavour and acidity for your taste receptors.

Finally, non-acidic fruit and vegetable juices provide a palatable remedy for anyone suffering from acid reflux. By including these beverages in your acid reflux cookbook, you may enjoy tasty and calming drinks without fear of provoking reflux symptoms. Cheers to a wonderful trip towards acid reflux cure!

Infused Water Recipes for Hydration

Infused water recipes offer a flavorful and refreshing way to stay hydrated while also providing relief for those experiencing acid reflux symptoms.

By infusing water with various fruits, herbs, and spices, you can create delicious beverages that not only quench your thirst but also soothe your digestive system. Here are some infused water recipes specifically tailored to provide relief for acid reflux:

Ginger and Lemon Infused Water:

Ingredients:

1. 1-inch piece of fresh ginger, thinly sliced
2. 1 lemon, thinly sliced 3. 4 cups of water
4. Instructions:
5. In a pitcher, combine the sliced ginger and lemon.
6. Fill the pitcher with water.
7. Refrigerate for at least 1 hour to allow the flavors to infuse.
8. Serve chilled over ice and enjoy the refreshing and soothing taste of ginger and lemon.

Cucumber and Mint Infused Water:

Ingredients:

1. 1 cucumber, thinly sliced
2. Handful of fresh mint leaves 3. 4 cups of water
4. Instructions:
5. Place the cucumber slices and mint leaves in a pitcher.
6. Add water to the pitcher.
7. Allow the mixture to infuse in the refrigerator for at least 1 hour.
8. Serve cold and revel in the cooling and calming effects of cucumber and mint.

Watermelon and Basil Infused Water:

Ingredients:

1. 1 cup of cubed watermelon
2. Handful of fresh basil leaves 3. 4 cups of water
4. Instructions:
5. In a pitcher, combine the cubed watermelon and basil leaves.

6. Pour water into the pitcher.
7. Refrigerate for at least 1 hour to infuse the flavors.
8. Serve chilled and delight in the sweet and herbaceous notes of watermelon and basil.

Lemon and Lavender Infused Water:

Ingredients:

1. 1 lemon, thinly sliced
2. 1 tablespoon of culinary lavender buds 3. 4 cups of water

Instructions:

4. Place the lemon slices and lavender buds in a pitcher.
5. Fill the pitcher with water.
6. Let the mixture sit in the refrigerator for at least 1 hour to infuse.
7. Serve cold and enjoy the subtle floral aroma and citrusy flavor of lemon and lavender.

These infused water recipes provide a tasty and hydrating alternative to sugary beverages, which can exacerbate acid reflux symptoms. Plus, they contain natural ingredients that may help alleviate discomfort and promote better digestion. Incorporate these refreshing beverages into your daily routine for a flavorful and soothing way to stay hydrated while managing acid reflux.

Chapter 6: Desserts and Treats for Acid Reflux

Banana Ice Cream

Ingredients:

1. 4 ripe bananas, peeled and sliced
2. 2 tablespoons honey or maple syrup (optional)
3. 1 teaspoon vanilla extract (optional)

Instructions:

1. Place the sliced bananas on a baking sheet lined with parchment paper.
2. Freeze the bananas for at least 2 hours or until solid.
3. Once frozen, transfer the bananas to a food processor or highpowered blender.
4. Add honey or maple syrup and vanilla extract, if using.
5. Blend the mixture until smooth and creamy, scraping down the sides of the processor or blender as needed.

6. Serve immediately for a soft-serve consistency or transfer to an airtight container and freeze for an additional 1-2 hours for a firmer texture.

7. Enjoy your delicious and creamy banana ice cream!

Nutritional Information:

1. Serving Size: 1/2 cup
2. Calories: 105
3. Total Fat: 0.3g
4. Saturated Fat: 0.1g
5. Cholesterol: 0mg
6. Sodium: 1mg
7. Total Carbohydrates: 27g
8. Dietary Fiber: 3.1g
9. Sugars: 14g
10. Protein: 1.2g

Cooking Time: 5 minutes preparation, 2 hours freezing

Baked Apples with Cinnamon

Ingredients:

1. 4 medium-sized apples (such as Granny Smith or Honeycrisp)
2. 2 tablespoons of honey or maple syrup
3. 1 teaspoon of ground cinnamon
4. 1/4 teaspoon of ground nutmeg
5. 1/4 cup of chopped pecans or walnuts (optional)
6. 1 tablespoon of unsalted butter or coconut oil, melted

Instructions:

1. Preheat your oven to 375°F (190°C).
2. Wash the apples thoroughly and then core them using an apple corer or a small knife, making sure to remove the seeds and stem but leaving the bottoms intact.
3. In a small bowl, mix together the honey or maple syrup, ground cinnamon, ground nutmeg, and chopped nuts (if using).
4. Place the cored apples in a baking dish, standing upright.
5. Spoon the honey-cinnamon mixture into the center of each apple, dividing it evenly among them.

6. Drizzle the melted butter or coconut oil over the top of each apple.

7. Bake the apples in the preheated oven for 30-40 minutes, or until they are tender and the skins start to wrinkle.

8. Remove the baked apples from the oven and let them cool slightly before serving.

Nutritional Information:

1. Serving Size: 1 baked apple
2. Calories: Approximately 120
3. Total Fat: 3g
4. Saturated Fat: 1g
5. Cholesterol: 5mg
6. Sodium: 0mg
7. Total Carbohydrates: 25g
8. Dietary Fiber: 4g
9. Sugars: 19g
10. Protein: 1g

Cooking Time: 30-40 minutes

Mango Coconut Chia Pudding

Ingredients:

1. 1 ripe mango, peeled and diced
2. 1 cup coconut milk
3. 1/4 cup chia seeds
4. 1 tablespoon honey or maple syrup (optional)
5. 1/2 teaspoon vanilla extract

Instructions:

1. In a blender, combine the diced mango, coconut milk, honey or maple syrup (if using), and vanilla extract. Blend until smooth.
2. Pour the mango coconut mixture into a mixing bowl.
3. Stir in the chia seeds until well combined.
4. Cover the bowl and refrigerate for at least 2 hours or overnight, allowing the chia seeds to expand and create a pudding-like consistency.
5. Before serving, give the pudding a good stir to distribute the chia seeds evenly.
6. Serve chilled, optionally garnished with additional diced mango or shredded coconut if desired.

Nutritional Information (per serving):

1. Calories: 220
2. Total Fat: 15g
3. Saturated Fat: 10g
4. Cholesterol: 0mg
5. Sodium: 20mg
6. Total Carbohydrates: 22g
7. Dietary Fiber: 6g
8. Sugars: 14g
9. Protein: 4g

Serving Size: 1/2 cup

Cooking Time: 2 hours chilling time

Chapter 7: Tips for Dining Out with Acid Reflux

Choosing Acid Reflux-Friendly Restaurants

When dining out with acid reflux, selecting the proper restaurant might help you manage your symptoms and enjoy your meal without suffering. Look for eateries that provide a choice of options for those with acid reflux.

Choose restaurants that prioritise fresh, whole foods and provide customisable menus to fit dietary constraints. Avoid places that serve heavy, oily food or spicy cuisine, as they might increase acid reflux symptoms.

Consider the restaurant's ambiance and environment. Choose a calmer, more comfortable environment where you may enjoy your lunch without feeling rushed or agitated.

Loud, crowded surroundings can add to indigestion and discomfort, so find a restaurant with a more relaxed ambiance that promotes digestion. When reading the menu, look for lighter, less acidic items that are easier on the stomach. Look for recipes containing lean meats, such as grilled chicken or fish, and lots of veggies. Avoid fried meals, creamy sauces, and high-fat dishes, as they might cause acid reflux symptoms.

Tell your server about your dietary needs and preferences. Request ingredient swaps or tweaks to make foods more acid reflux friendly. Most restaurants are happy to accommodate specific requests, so do not be afraid to speak up and fight for your health.

When ordering, be aware of portion proportions.

Overeating can put strain on the stomach and worsen acid reflux symptoms. To avoid overeating, order smaller servings or share meals with your dining mates.

Choose beverages sensibly, preferring water or herbal tea over alcohol or fizzy beverages, which can cause acid reflux. If you do want to consume alcohol, do it in moderation and avoid beverages with strong acidity, such as citrus-based cocktails.

Finally, listen to your body and see how various meals impact your symptoms. If you are experiencing pain after a meal, keep track of everything you ate and how it was cooked. Over time, you will discover which meals and places are ideal for treating acid reflux, allowing you to make more educated dining decisions.

Strategies for Ordering Acid Reflux-Friendly Meals

When dining out with acid reflux, it is critical to use tactics that prioritise your digestive health while also enjoying wonderful meals.

Familiarising oneself with the menu ahead of time is a smart method. Many restaurants provide online menus, which allows you to plan ahead of time and find acid reflux-friendly selections.

Look for foods reduced in fat and spices, as these might worsen reflux symptoms. In addition, choosing lean meats such as grilled chicken or fish, as well as vegetables and nutritious grains, might help reduce pain.

Another crucial tip for selecting acid reflux-friendly dishes while eating out is to convey your dietary requirements to the restaurant's personnel. Don't be afraid to ask inquiries about how foods are made and seek changes to meet your condition. For example, you might request that sauces and dressings be served on the side or replaced with options that are less likely to cause reflux. Most restaurants will accommodate specific dietary demands, so don't be hesitant to fight for your health.

When reviewing the menu, choose basic, plain foods over elaborate or excessively seasoned ones. Plain grilled or baked foods are frequently safer than dishes with thick sauces or strong spices. Additionally, choosing smaller serving sizes might help prevent overeating, which can exacerbate acid symptoms. Consider splitting a meal with a dining buddy or ordering appetisers as your main dish to keep portion proportions under control and avoid discomfort later.

When dining out with acid reflux, it's also a good idea to choose your beverages carefully. Certain beverages, such as citrus juices, carbonated drinks, and alcohol, might worsen reflux symptoms.

Instead, choose water, herbal teas, or non-citrus fruit juices as more calming options. If you prefer to consume alcohol, do it in moderation and avoid very acidic or carbonated beverages.

When dining out, be proactive in minimising your GERD symptoms by adopting mindful eating practices. Take your time chewing your food completely and savouring each bite, as speeding through meals increases the probability of reflux. Also, pay attention to how different meals influence your body and establish a list of any triggers you should avoid in the future. Staying attentive to your body's cues allows you to make more educated mealtime decisions.

When dining out with acid reflux, consider not just what you eat but also when you consume it. Eating smaller, more frequent meals throughout the day can assist to avoid overloading your digestive system and lessen the chance of acid symptoms. Avoid eating heavy meals late at night, as laying down soon after eating might worsen reflux. Instead, dine early in the evening and give yourself plenty of time to digest before going to bed.

Finally, don't be afraid to carry any drugs or solutions you use to treat your acid reflux symptoms when dining out. Having them on available can bring peace of mind and guarantee that you are ready to deal with any pain that may develop. Consider taking antacids or other over-the-counter medicines with you to provide extra relief in the event of a sudden flare-up. By applying these measures and being proactive about your food choices, you may enjoy eating out while reducing the impact of acid reflux on your digestive health.

Handling Social Situations and Special Occasions

Navigating social events and special occasions while suffering from acid reflux can be difficult. However, with proper preparation and observation, you can still eat out without exacerbating your symptoms. Here are some suggestions to help you handle eating out with acid reflux:

1. **Choose Wisely:** Before visiting a restaurant, look out their menu online. Look for selections with less fat and acidity, as they might worsen acid reflux symptoms. Choose grilled, roasted, or steamed foods over fried or overly sauced options.

2. **Be Mindful of Portions:** Restaurant servings are frequently greater than what you would normally consume at home. To avoid overeating, consider splitting an entree or ordering a half serving.

3. **Modify Your Order:** Don't be afraid to ask your waiter whether some meals may be cooked without elements known to cause acid reflux, such as onions, garlic, tomatoes, or spicy spices. Many restaurants accommodate dietary restrictions and can make replacements or adaptations to meet your needs.

4. **Avoid Trigger Foods:** Identify your own trigger foods and avoid them when eating out. Acid reflux is commonly triggered by citrus fruits, chocolate, coffee, mint, and alcohol. Be aware of the hidden sources of these components in sauces, dressings, and marinades.

5. **Eat Slowly and Mindfully:** Take your time to chew your food thoroughly and savor each bite. Eating too quickly can lead to overeating and indigestion. Additionally, be mindful of your portion sizes and stop eating when you feel comfortably full to prevent discomfort and reflux symptoms.

6. **Stay Hydrated:** Opt for water or non-acidic beverages like herbal tea instead of carbonated drinks, which

can increase gastric pressure and contribute to reflux. Drinking plenty of water throughout your meal can help dilute stomach acid and promote digestion.

7. **Practice Good Posture:** Sit upright while eating to prevent pressure on your stomach and minimize the risk of acid reflux. Avoid slouching or lying down immediately after a meal, as this can exacerbate symptoms.

8. **Consider Timing:** Plan your dining out experience during times when you're less likely to experience reflux symptoms. Avoid eating too close to bedtime, as lying down shortly after a meal can increase the likelihood of acid reflux. Aim to eat at least two to three hours before going to bed.

9. **Bring Medication:** If you regularly take medication for acid reflux, make sure to bring it with you when dining out. Take your medication as prescribed, and don't wait until symptoms appear before taking it.

10. **Listen to Your Body:** Pay attention to how your body reacts to different foods and environments when dining out. If certain restaurants or types of cuisine consistently trigger your acid reflux symptoms, consider exploring alternative dining options or preparing meals at home more frequently.

By following these tips and being proactive about managing your acid reflux, you can enjoy dining out with confidence and without discomfort. Remember to prioritize your health and well-being while still savoring the social aspects of sharing meals with friends and loved ones.

Chapter 8: Lifestyle Changes for Managing Acid Reflux

Tips for Improving Digestion and Reducing Stress

Improving digestion and reducing stress are two crucial components of managing acid reflux effectively. By adopting certain lifestyle changes, individuals can alleviate symptoms and improve their overall well-being. Here are some tips to enhance digestion and minimize stress, which can significantly contribute to managing acid reflux:

1. Mindful Eating:

Practicing mindful eating involves being fully present during meals, paying attention to hunger cues, and savoring each bite. Chew food slowly and thoroughly to aid digestion and prevent overeating, which can exacerbate acid reflux symptoms. Avoid eating on the go or while distracted, as this can lead to poor digestion and increased stress on the digestive system.

2. Maintain a Healthy Weight:

Excess weight can put pressure on the stomach and increase the risk of acid reflux. By maintaining a healthy weight through a balanced diet and regular exercise, individuals can reduce the severity and frequency of reflux episodes. Focus on consuming nutrient-dense foods and engaging in physical activity that you enjoy to support weight management and overall health.

3. Eat Smaller, More Frequent Meals:

Large meals can trigger acid reflux symptoms due to increased stomach pressure. Instead of consuming three large meals per day, opt for smaller, more frequent meals to prevent overloading the digestive system. Eating smaller portions can help reduce the likelihood of acid reflux and promote better digestion. Be mindful of portion sizes and avoid eating late at night, which can disrupt sleep and exacerbate reflux symptoms.

4. Identify Trigger Foods:

Certain foods and beverages can exacerbate acid reflux symptoms in susceptible individuals. Common triggers include spicy foods, citrus fruits, caffeine, alcohol, and high-fat meals. Keep a food diary to identify specific triggers and minimize their consumption. Experiment with eliminating or reducing trigger foods from your diet to determine their impact on acid reflux symptoms. Focus on incorporating more alkaline-forming foods, such as leafy greens, vegetables, and whole grains, to support digestive health.

5. Manage Stress:

Stress can worsen acid reflux symptoms by increasing stomach acid production and altering digestive processes. Incorporate stress-reducing activities into your daily routine, such as meditation, yoga, deep breathing exercises, or spending time in nature. Prioritize self-care and relaxation to minimize stress levels and promote overall well-being. Establishing a regular sleep schedule and practicing good sleep hygiene can also help reduce stress and improve digestive function.

6. Stay Hydrated:

Proper hydration is essential for maintaining optimal digestive health. Drink plenty of water throughout the day to support digestion, prevent dehydration, and dilute stomach acid. Limit consumption of carbonated beverages, sugary drinks, and caffeinated beverages, as they can contribute to acid reflux symptoms. Herbal teas, such as ginger or chamomile tea, may have soothing effects on the digestive system and help alleviate discomfort associated with acid reflux.

7. Practice Good Posture:

Poor posture can contribute to acid reflux by putting pressure on the abdomen and interfering with digestion. Maintain good posture while sitting, standing, and walking to support proper digestion and reduce the risk of reflux. Avoid slouching or lying down immediately after eating, as this can worsen symptoms. Use pillows to elevate the head and upper body while sleeping to prevent acid from refluxing into the esophagus.

By implementing these lifestyle changes, individuals can improve digestion, reduce stress, and effectively manage acid reflux symptoms. Consistency and patience are key, as it may take time to notice significant improvements. Experiment with different strategies to find what works best for you and consult with a healthcare professional for personalized guidance and support.

Incorporating Exercise into Your Routine

Incorporating exercise into your routine is a crucial aspect of managing acid reflux and promoting overall well-being. Regular physical activity not only helps in maintaining a healthy weight, but it also aids in reducing symptoms of acid reflux by improving digestion, reducing stress, and strengthening the muscles that support the lower esophageal sphincter (LES), which helps prevent stomach acid from flowing back into the esophagus.

When it comes to choosing the right type of exercise for acid reflux management, it's essential to opt for activities that are lowimpact and unlikely to trigger reflux symptoms. Activities such as walking, cycling, swimming, and gentle yoga are excellent choices as they promote relaxation and improve circulation without putting excessive strain on the digestive system.

It's important to note that while exercise is beneficial for acid reflux, timing is key. Engaging in vigorous exercise immediately after a meal can exacerbate symptoms by putting pressure on the stomach and causing stomach acid to reflux into the esophagus. Therefore, it's advisable to wait at least two to three hours after eating before engaging in intense physical activity.

Incorporating exercise into your daily routine doesn't have to be complicated or time-consuming. Even small changes such as taking the stairs instead of the elevator, parking farther away from your destination to get in some extra steps, or incorporating short walks into your lunch break can make a significant difference in managing acid reflux symptoms and improving overall health.

Consistency is key when it comes to reaping the benefits of exercise for acid reflux management. Aim for at least 30 minutes of moderate-intensity exercise most days of the week, and gradually increase the duration and intensity as your fitness level improves. Remember to listen to your body and choose activities that you enjoy and are sustainable in the long term.

In addition to incorporating regular physical activity into your routine, it's also important to pay attention to your posture during exercise. Poor posture can put added pressure on the abdomen, leading to increased risk of acid reflux. Focus on maintaining good posture, especially during exercises that involve bending or twisting motions, and consider incorporating exercises that strengthen the muscles of the core and back to support proper alignment.

In conclusion, incorporating exercise into your routine is an essential component of managing acid reflux and promoting overall health. By choosing low-impact activities, timing your workouts appropriately, and maintaining good posture, you can effectively reduce symptoms of acid reflux and improve your quality of life. Remember to consult with your healthcare provider before starting any new exercise regimen, especially if you have pre-existing medical conditions.

Getting Quality Sleep to Prevent Acid Reflux Episodes

Getting quality sleep is crucial for managing acid reflux effectively. Poor sleep can exacerbate symptoms and increase the frequency of acid reflux episodes. In Chapter 8 of the Acid Reflux Cookbook, we delve into the importance of lifestyle changes, particularly focusing on how improving sleep habits can prevent acid reflux episodes.

Quality sleep is essential for overall health and well-being, and it plays a significant role in managing acid reflux. When you don't get enough sleep or experience poor sleep quality, it can lead to a range of issues that may worsen acid reflux symptoms. Research has shown that insufficient sleep can contribute to increased acid production in the stomach and a weakened lower esophageal sphincter (LES), which can result in acid reflux.

Several strategies can help you achieve better sleep and reduce the likelihood of acid reflux episodes. First and foremost, it's essential to establish a consistent sleep schedule by going to bed and waking up at the same time every day, even on weekends. This helps regulate your body's internal clock, promoting better sleep quality and minimizing disruptions to your digestive system.

Creating a relaxing bedtime routine can also promote better sleep and reduce acid reflux symptoms. This may include activities such as reading, taking a warm bath, or practicing relaxation techniques like deep breathing or meditation. Avoiding stimulating activities and electronic devices close to bedtime can help signal to your body that it's time to wind down and prepare for sleep.

Maintaining a comfortable sleep environment is another key factor in preventing acid reflux episodes. Sleeping on your left side or with your upper body elevated can help reduce the likelihood of acid reflux by keeping stomach acid from flowing back into the esophagus. Investing in a supportive mattress and pillows can also improve sleep quality and reduce discomfort associated with acid reflux.

In addition to these strategies, it's important to be mindful of your dietary choices and eating habits, as these can significantly impact both sleep quality and acid reflux symptoms. Avoiding large meals, spicy or acidic foods, and caffeine close to bedtime can help prevent nighttime reflux and promote better sleep. It's also advisable to limit alcohol consumption, as it can relax the LES and contribute to acid reflux.

In conclusion, prioritizing quality sleep is essential for managing acid reflux and preventing symptoms from worsening. By incorporating healthy sleep habits and making lifestyle changes, such as maintaining a consistent sleep schedule, creating a relaxing bedtime routine, and optimizing your sleep environment, you can reduce the frequency and severity of acid reflux episodes, leading to improved overall health and well-being.

30 DAYS MEAL PLAN

Day	Breakfast	Lunch	Dinner	Snack
1	Oatmeal with Bananas and Almonds	Greek Yogurt Parfait with Berries	Egg White Veggie Omelet	Quinoa Salad with Grilled Chicken
2	Greek Yogurt Parfait with Berries	Egg White Veggie Omelet	Quinoa Salad with Grilled Chicken	Turkey and Avocado Wrap
3	Egg White Veggie Omelet	Quinoa Salad with Grilled Chicken	Turkey and Avocado Wrap	Salmon and Vegetable Stir-Fry
4	Quinoa Salad with Grilled Chicken	Turkey and Avocado Wrap	Salmon and Vegetable Stir-Fry	Baked Chicken Breast with Roasted Vegetables
5	Turkey and Avocado Wrap	Salmon and Vegetable Stir-Fry	Baked Chicken Breast with Roasted Vegetables	Shrimp and Vegetable Skewers

Day	Breakfast	Lunch	Dinner	Snack
...	...	...	...	...
28	Banana Ice Cream	Baked Apples with Cinnamon	Mango Coconut Chia Pudding	Oatmeal with Bananas and Almonds
29	Baked Apples with Cinnamon	Mango Coconut Chia Pudding	Oatmeal with Bananas and Almonds	Greek Yogurt Parfait with Berries
30	Mango Coconut Chia Pudding	Oatmeal with Bananas and Almonds	Greek Yogurt Parfait with Berries	Egg White Veggie Omelet

Conclusion

In conclusion, the Acid Reflux Cookbook offers a comprehensive guide to managing acid reflux through dietary changes, lifestyle adjustments, and healthy habits. Throughout the cookbook, we have explored the role of various foods in triggering or alleviating acid reflux symptoms, providing readers with a wealth of delicious and nutritious recipes that promote digestive health and reduce discomfort.

By emphasizing the importance of a balanced diet rich in whole grains, fruits, vegetables, lean proteins, and healthy fats, the cookbook empowers individuals to make informed choices that support their overall well-being and minimize the risk of acid reflux flare-ups. By incorporating anti-inflammatory ingredients, such as ginger, turmeric, and leafy greens, into their meals, readers can help reduce inflammation in the digestive tract and alleviate symptoms associated with acid reflux.

Furthermore, the cookbook highlights the significance of lifestyle modifications in managing acid reflux effectively. From practicing mindful eating and portion control to adopting strategies for stress management and improving sleep quality, readers are encouraged to take a holistic approach to managing their condition. By addressing underlying factors that contribute to acid reflux, such as obesity, smoking, and sedentary behavior, individuals can enhance the effectiveness of dietary interventions and experience long-term relief from symptoms.

In addition to offering practical tips and recipes, the Acid Reflux Cookbook emphasizes the importance of personalized care and ongoing support in managing acid reflux. While dietary changes and lifestyle modifications play a central role in symptom management, it is essential for individuals to work closely with healthcare professionals to develop a comprehensive treatment plan tailored to their unique needs and preferences.

Overall, the Acid Reflux Cookbook serves as a valuable resource for individuals seeking to take control of their acid reflux and improve their quality of life. By empowering readers with knowledge, practical tools, and delicious recipes, the cookbook equips them with the resources they need to make positive changes and achieve lasting relief from acid reflux symptoms. Whether you are newly diagnosed with acid reflux or have been managing the condition for years, the Acid Reflux Cookbook offers guidance and inspiration to support you on your journey to better digestive health.

www.ingramcontent.com/pod-product-compliance
Lightning Source LLC
Chambersburg PA
CBHW050326230526
45471CB00005B/2373